Quarto.com

© 2024 Quarto Publishing Group
USA Inc.

First Published in 2024 by Fair Winds
Press, an imprint of The Quarto Group,
100 Cummings Center, Suite 265-D,
Beverly, MA 01915, USA.
T (978) 282-9590 F (978) 283-2742

Fair Winds Press titles are also available
at discount for retail, wholesale,
promotional, and bulk purchase.
For details, contact the Special Sales
Manager by email at specialsales@
quarto.com or by mail at The Quarto
Group, Attn: Special Sales Manager, 100
Cummings Center, Suite 265-D, Beverly,
MA 01915, USA.

28 27 26 25 24   1 2 3 4 5

ISBN: 978-0-7603-9244-7

Digital edition published in 2024
eISBN: 978-0-7603-9245-4

Library of Congress Cataloging-in-
Publication Data

Names: Hamilton, Jill, editor, compiler.
Title: Steamy sex games / compiled and
edited by Jill Hamilton.
Description: Beverly, MA : Fair Winds
Press, an imprint of The Quarto
   Group, 2024. | Series: The erotic
couple's playbook | Summary: "Steamy
   Sex Games adds spice to your sex life
with dozens of tantalizing
   seductions and scenarios"-- Provided
by publisher.
Identifiers: LCCN 2024018313 | ISBN
9780760392447 (hardcover) | ISBN
   9780760392454 (ebook)
Subjects: LCSH: Sex.
Classification: LCC HQ21 .S628 2024 |
DDC 306.77--dc23/eng/20240508
LC record available at https://lccn.loc.
gov/202

Compiled and edited by Jill Hamilton
Design and layout: Burge Agency
Illustration: Sandra Alutyte

Printed in Hong Kong

The information in this book is for
educational purposes only. Any type of
sexual activity should be consensual.

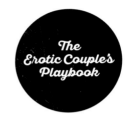

The
Erotic Couple's
Playbook

Steamy
Sex
Games

QUIVER

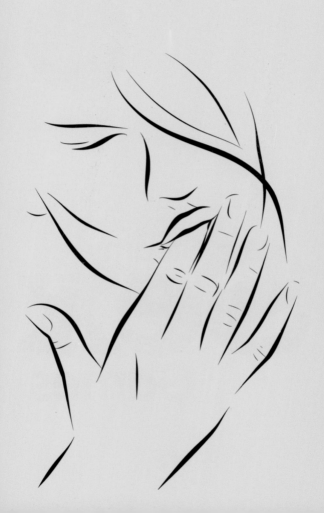

Contents

How to Use This Book

These sex games are designed to bring you closer and give your sex life all the fire emojis. Bust out this book whenever you want to zhuzh up your sex life and make yourselves insane with lust for each other. If everyone's hard/wet and in need of an orgasm at the end—congratulations!—you have won that game.

Store this book in your nightstand, take it with you on a weekend getaway, stow it away, or give it to your partner as a surprise. You can pick out a game together or be very brave and open to a random page to let fate decide what you will try.

There are an array of games in here, from silly to sexy to semi-kinky, and if there's one that sounds funky to you, don't do it! No points deducted. *But* if there's a little part of you that wants to try something that seems semi-jacked-up, maybe give it a go. You might find your new favorite thing.

Let the games begin.

Strip Poker

01

The OG sex game

Instead of just getting naked with no fanfare, add some drama with a competitive game of strip poker. In the classic version, the loser of each hand must remove an article of clothing.

You'll be playing seven-card stud. Deal two cards face down and one card face up. Make a bet (e.g., fifty cents, one dollar, etc.), then deal three cards face up and the final card face down. Winning hands (highest to lowest) are as follows: royal flush, straight flush, flush, full house, three of a kind, two pair, one pair. One pair beats the highest card in the hand.

Decide beforehand who—winner or loser—will decide what comes off. Keep playing as long as you can stand it—it's kind of hard to concentrate on remembering if three of a kind beats two pairs when one or both of you is right there all fetchingly naked.

If you want to up the ante, the winner of each hand gets to command the loser to perform a service like "massage my feet," "kiss every inch of my boobs," or "suck on the tip of my penis for a minute." Go as hardcore as you want, as long as you've agreed on boundaries before you start the game. (When you veer into the more kinky stuff, it's kind of like childhood Monopoly games—way better if you figure out the rules beforehand.)

01

Bonus tip! Make strip versions of whatever you want. Strip Boggle? Strip Wii Bowling? Bring it on!

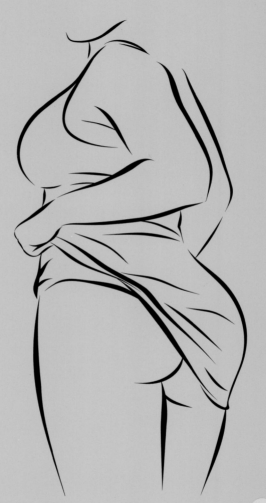

Naked Wrestling

02

It's like mud wrestling, without the mud

Harness the primitive appeal of mud wrestling with your own at-home version. Getting wet, slippery, and sliding all over each other, is not just plenty fun, but the competition and pretend danger boosts your adrenaline, which makes you feel more attached to each other. (It's science!)

To get those good chemicals flowing, throw down a bunch of old towels or blankets. The floor is better than a bed because this is gonna be messy, but if you prep *extremely* well, a bed can work, too. Put down a plastic sheet or even some garbage bags under the blanket/towels if you want to be extra careful. There are also special sex blankets you can buy for messy stuff like this.

Cover yourselves in *tons* of lube and try to pin each other down. You can just embrace the general hotness of rubbing against each other or make actual rules. Try a submission round where the person who gives in does what the victor says. Keep the commands short to keep it going and maximize arousal, like "stroke my cock/vulva for one minute" or "spread your legs for me and touch yourself until I tell you to stop."

If it gets too intense—and it absolutely can feel that way to be pinned and helpless—have a safe word to stop the action immediately.

02

Bonus tip! For another version, each of you tries to remove an item of clothing from the other person.

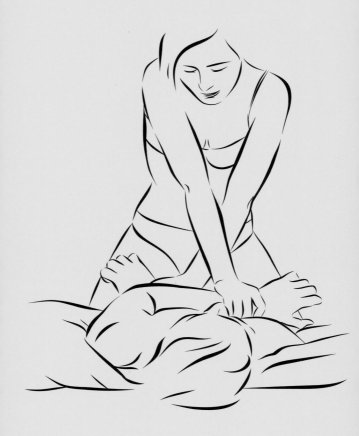

How Long Can You Last?

03

What will win out— competition or pure lust?

Watching your partner succumb to the overwhelming force that is an inevitable orgasm is already pretty hot, but watching them succumb while they're actively trying *not* to come adds a whole extra level of intriguing mental f*ckery. Especially when you are the one causing them to go over the edge.

See how much resolve your partner has by having them read aloud from a book, instructing them to continue as long as they can. It can be any book—a classic novel, a textbook on economics, whatever. While they read, start stimulating them with your hands, mouth, or a favorite toy. See how long they can keep it together. Their challenge? Keep reading without just giving up, throwing the book down, and submitting to your sexual superpowers.

Your challenge? Do everything you can to make them lose their sh*t (not literally) and give into the glory of your mouth/hands/toy.

Make it more competitive by raising the stakes. If you partner can't get through a certain number of pages without having to stop, then they must do your sexual bidding. Or if they do somehow make it through the pages (impossible!), you have to do their sexual bidding.

If your partner is stubborn and/or you want to make it harder on them, switch out the neutral reading materials with some erotica that you know does it for them.

03

Bonus tip! For a variation, go visual. Have them go through a series of new dirty photos of you or watch a favorite porn, describing what they see.

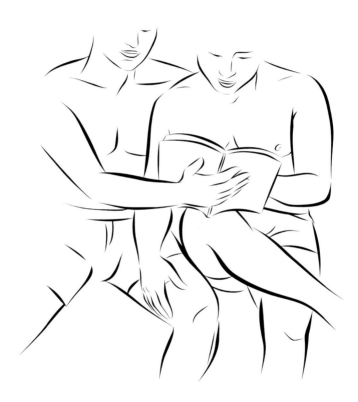

Private Cam Performer

04

Let the show begin

Set aside some time for a *very* personal FaceTime session where one of you will be the other's sex cam performer.

If you're the cam performer, play it up. Use a low sexy voice and flirt with the camera. Bust out the silky lingerie, the leather chaps, or whatever it is that makes you feel sexy and hot. Outfit your space so it looks sexy by lighting some candles and putting on some quiet music in the background. Let your client tell you what they'd like to see. If they just want to watch you, take your time teasing them. Take your clothes off piece by piece, talking about what you're doing. Or lie back in the bed and start slowly touching yourself.

If you're the client, go ahead and indulge your fantasies. Maybe you'd like to indulge in a voyeuristic fantasy where your cam performer is doing a strip tease just for you. Or maybe you'd like to give them very explicit instructions like "open your legs for me" or "start stroking your cock so I can watch."

Go ahead and play with personas, too, if you'd like. It works for both sides of the camera. Maybe the cam performer is a dominatrix barking instructions to her client that must be obeyed. Take it wherever you want. It's y'all's fantasy: No one needs to know what happens between you.

04

Bonus tip! This absolutely works as a live, in-person performance, too.

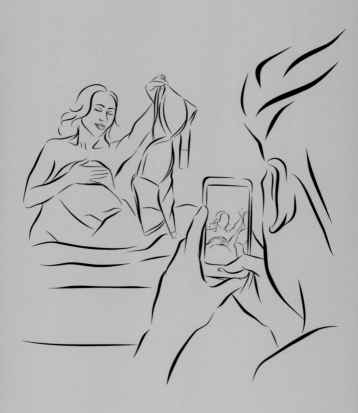

Screen Test

05

Role-play with a script

Is there a scene from a movie or TV show that really turns you on? A sexy thriller? An epic romance? Everything about *Bridgerton*? Reenact it! Start by rewatching the scene to "study" it. What makes it sexy to you? The setting? The particular way an actor bites their lip? A position you'd like to try?

Be as faithful to the source material as you'd like. If you like a sex scene in a shower, maybe just having sex in the shower will do the trick. If you want to recreate the scene shot-by-shot, that's cool, too. You can choreograph the moves and copy them exactly. And, if you want to add more role-play into it, go full method actor. Come to the scene as your characters and have sex as the characters. Be as extra as you want. Wear a costume, decorate the "set" in the style of the movie, play the same song in the background. Say the lines verbatim if you want (if there are any—it *is* a sex scene).

For an extra level of veracity and hotness, film it. Use your own camera and make some revenge porn. And yes, seeing your bare butts grinding away in full detail without the services of a professional cinematographer can be an un-fun reality check on how much your romp did *not*, in fact, resemble the actual movie. However, you two look like you which is even better because it's 100% real.

05

Bonus tip! Play the scene as you're reenacting it for inspiration/ reminders of what you're supposed to be doing.

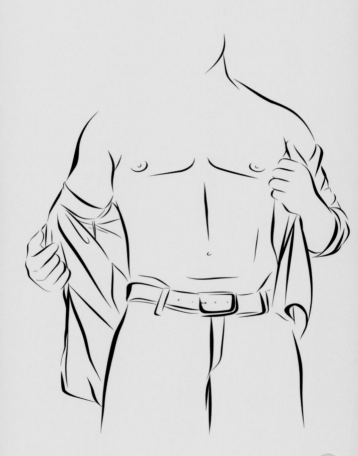

Extra Whip, Please

06

All you can eat

Yes, using food as a part of sex has such a "ye olde women's magazine sex tip"-vibe. And yet, both food and sex are about sensual pleasure and, if you can enjoy both at once, all the better!

The recipe is easy: you squirt, your partner licks. Take a can of whipped cream and put a dollop somewhere you'd like to be licked. Guide your partner around your body via whipped cream. Squirt a puffy cloud of cream on each nipple. Trail a line up your inner thigh. Squirt a dab on the end of your tongue and have them suck it off.

Adjust your choice of sexy food according to taste. If canned whipped cream is not your thing, try chocolate syrup or honey. Pretty much anything works as long as it's not something that's going to irritate your skin and it's something that your partner is willing to consume a decent amount of. (This is why edible lube isn't such a great option. Even though it's edible, it doesn't mean that anyone actually wants to snack on it.) And keep all food stuff out of the vagina. Outside on the vulva is A-OK. Inside is no bueno.

After you are both fully sated with food and sex, a nice way to finish is by slipping into the shower together and lathering all that debauchery off of each other.

06

**Bonus tip!
For a less messy
taste-fest, you
can use non-
liquid things
like berries
or chocolate
candies.**

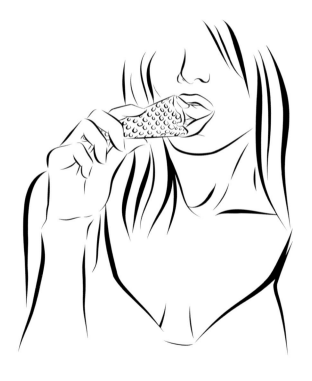

You Actually ARE the Boss of Me

07

You will be mine

Take your partner on as your personal sex slave. As the master/mistress or Dominant, you will set the agenda and take charge.

What will you do with your vast powers? You could order the Sub to touch themselves to your specifications while you watch. You could insist upon oral on demand. You could make them strip for you. Your wish is their command.

If you want to kink it up, go further with the BDSM aspects. Insist that your partner call you by your Dom name like Master or Mistress. Give your Sub a pet name—okay if it's semi-humiliating, that's part of it. Give your Sub tasks and praise them lavishly if they please you, and punish them if they don't.

Set up all the rules beforehand so that once you're in the experience you can both relax into it and feel safe. Create a safe word so that if someone needs to bail, it will happen immediately. Talk about expectations and boundaries. Is it okay to use restraints? Will physical punishment be allowed? Is humiliation okay or nah?

A Dom/Sub experience is intense and that can be overwhelming. Practice good aftercare by loving up your Sub afterward. Talk it over (yes, again! Lots of talking is important with BDSM and BDSM-adjacent sex) to process the experience. And if it all went well, plan the next one.

07

**Bonus tip!
If one of you
tends to be the
more dominant
one, switch
the dynamics
by having
them take the
submissive role.**

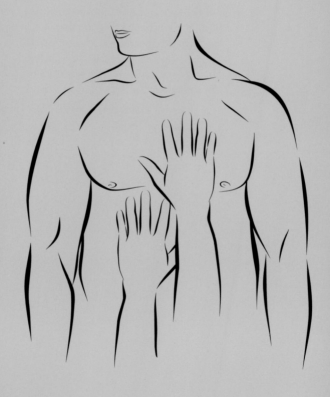

XXX Marco Polo

08

Dive on in

If you have access to a private pool or hot tub, invite your partner for a late-night game of Marco Polo. To play, your partner closes their eyes and seeks out your body in the water. You can play the traditional version: Your partner says "Marco" then you reply "Polo" and they can make their way to you based on where your voice sounds like it's coming from. Or you can porn it up: they call your name and you reply with a moan.

When they find you, reward them by pulling them close for a kiss, some underwater groping, or a bit of whispered dirty talk. Then switch roles and try to find them and claim your reward.

If the pool or hot tub is REALLY private, you have options: Strip out of your bathing suits. Try to jump up on a floating toy—and stay up—for a make-out session at sea. Sit on the top rung of the ladder for poolside oral.

Don't expect to use the water as lube unless chafing is your kink. Water is inexplicably drying in this situation so use lube for penetrative sex and all manner of handies.

If you're going for penetrative sex, next to the pool is better than in the pool. Try it with one person sitting on the edge of the pool or standing in the shallow end. Or, f*ck it (no pun intended), and just wrap up in some towels and take it to a poolside chaise lounge.

Bonus tip! Since water is weirdly drying down below, bring plenty of lube along. Use a silicone type that will last longer in water.

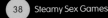

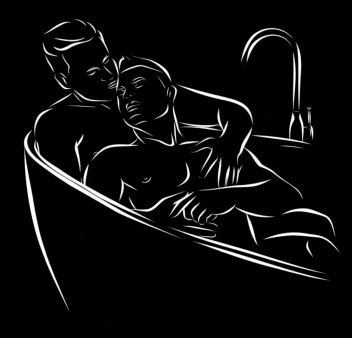

Espresso-Charged Quickie

09

I'll have a Venti, please

Caffeinate a regular old day with a stealthy
coffee shop rendezvous. Doing something a
little jacked up and daring together releases
the bonding chemical, oxytocin, which makes
y'all feel more in L-O-V-E, but it's also just fun.

Here's what gonna go down: Stake out
a good coffee house that's convenient to
both of you. Plan to arrive separately at the
designated time. Order and sit at separate
tables, pretending not to know each other.
A little flirty eye contact is allowed but keep it
to a minimum—acting like you're complete
strangers makes it even better.

When the time seems right, one of you heads into the restroom and the other waits a couple of minutes, then sneaks back to the same bathroom. Once you're both in, lock the door—then check to make sure that yes, it *is* super locked (repeat as needed)—then ravish each other. Try hiking a leg up on the toilet for standing penetration, oral while leaning against the sink, or mutual hand jobs.

This game makes a great workday nooner, especially since you can send each other important planning texts to build anticipation.

Here's how to make it great: stash a bottle of lube and bring it with you. Scope out your location beforehand to make sure bathrooms are large, clean and—important!—single occupancy. And if someone knocks, don't be a dick, get out and let them have the room.

09

Bonus tip! Have a secret knock so you're not knocking on some rando's bathroom door.

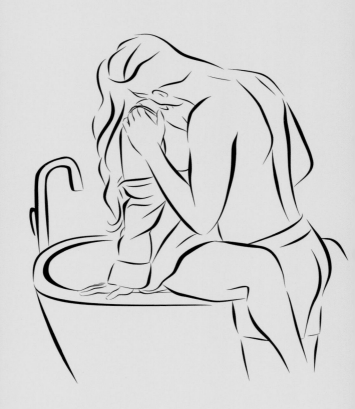

The All-Nighter

10

F*ck all night, sorta

To start this game, hop in bed at night and get each other well turned on, but not so much that you get to a point of no return. Stop, then kiss and cuddle, allowing yourselves to fall asleep in each other's arms in a semi-aroused haze.

As you wake in the night, try a few lazy thrusts or stroke each other with mutual handies. Don't linger too long with it: The idea is to stay in a state of mild arousal throughout the whole night. Sleepy, half-awake touching is what you're aiming for. Stay connected and aware of each other throughout the night, but not so turned on that it's going to keep you awake.

Trying this with penetration can be amazing. Few things are as intimate as falling asleep with one of you inside the other's ass or vagina. But if you're going in, a few things to know: If you're using a dildo, use something soft and flexible for more comfort for the receiving ass/vagina. And if a penis is involved, it will get soft in the night. Totally normal. Sweet lazy thrusts with a soft cock work too. Just be aware that a regular condom will slip off, so if you need protection from STIs or pregnancy, use a female condom instead.

In the morning, all bets are off. Go ahead and ravish each other. You know you want to.

10

Bonus tip! Use a long-lasting lube-like silicone that will stay slippery longer. Keep the bottle next to the bed so you can reapply.

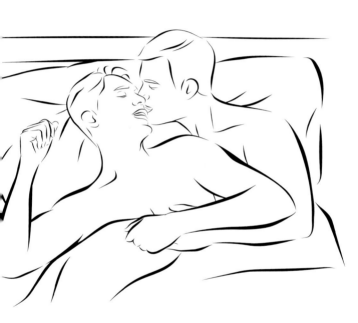

Like a Virgin

11

Touched for the very first time

For many among us, the actual experience of losing your virginity was not so great. So give yourselves a do over without the fumbling, awkwardness, and possible bad hair of the real first time by pretending you've never done IT before. (PSA: "Virginity" is a social construct. And "losing" it doesn't need to mean P-in-V. Define IT however you damn well please.)

Pretend you are both new to sex and have never touched each other. Take your time exploring each other's bodies and letting yourself be awed by what you uncover with each new removal of a piece of clothing or the feel of someone's lips between your legs for the pseudo first time.

You can add some drama by pretending what you're doing is so very forbidden—what if someone finds out!?—but you cannot stop yourselves. You could pretend to be different people entirely. Or you can just use the game as a chance to experience each other anew.

Trying something different—pretty much anything different—is a great way for you both to lock into the experience and each other. And that kind of focused attention is what really great sex is about. If you feel kind of skittish about full-on role-play, this is kind of a beginner version. No costumes, no characters necessary—just you and your partner rediscovering each other.

11

Bonus tip! Change the vibe by having one person pretend to be the experienced one who is teaching the other.

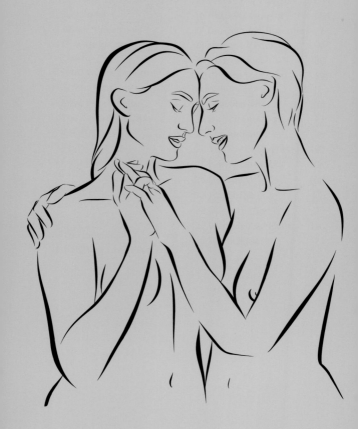

Aural Sex

12

Mmmmmmmm

There's an intensely intimate level of communication that takes place between lovers during sex: the whole private language of the sounds we make to each other. A deep moan of pleasure, a moment of desperate panting, your name rasped out in pleasure—these sounds are primal, deeply personal, and exclusive to sex. (No one makes these sounds at the gas station. Or at least not generally.)

Put the focus on these direct messages from the heart and groin by making a rule that you can't talk during sex. You must communicate entirely though sounds. See if you can let your partner know what you're feeling though the sounds you make. Softly sigh into their ear. Murmur approvingly as you lick a nipple. Allow a deep groan to escape your lips as they take you in their mouth. Let yourself freestyle incoherent sounds as you get closer to orgasm.

Go ahead and amp up the volume. Exaggerate your sounds so that your partner knows exactly what they're doing to you and how much you're into it and them. The more you convey what you're feeling through your moans, deep sighs, and heavy panting, the hotter it is.

To add an extra layer, allow yourselves one word each: the other person's name. Few things are headier than hearing someone in the throes who is moaning, whispering, sighing, and hell, maybe screaming your name.

12

**Bonus tip!
Try it during
phone sex.
No words,
just moans.**

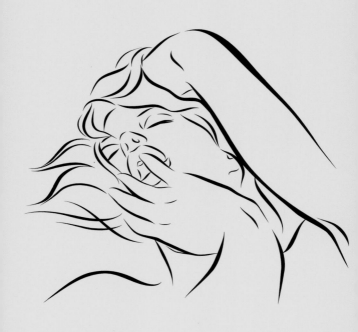

The Home Run

13

And the crowd goes wild

Remember the old base system of sex? First
base is kissing, second is boobs, third is
touching under the underwear, and a home
run was "going all the way." Traditionally, this
home run/all the way business meant penis
in vagina intercourse, but go ahead and
make it mean whatever you want it to mean.
Outercourse, oral, toys—whatever you two do
to give each other orgasms can be a homer.

Enlist the base system to have sex all over the
house, designating certain rooms for each
base. Start with a make out session in the
living room. Score! First base! Move to the

kitchen for second base, boobs! Since the base system was ill-defined on what happened here, probably feeling someone up, make this base your own. Do all the feeling up you want, plus kiss, lick, and suck on nipples. And don't forget that most people like nipple play, whether they're sporting lady boobs or moobs.

As you round over to third base, take turns sitting your asses up on the dining table and serve up tableside hand jobs or play with each other with toys. For the grand finale, head to the bedroom to hit a home run with orgasms for all, however you two like to get there. Afterwards, slap each other on the butt and hit the showers together. You played a good game.

**Bonus tip!
Put a special item
in each room
for each base.
Try painting
each other's lips
with syrup or
honey for first,
nipple clamps for
second, a vibrator
for third, and a
massage candle for
the home run.**

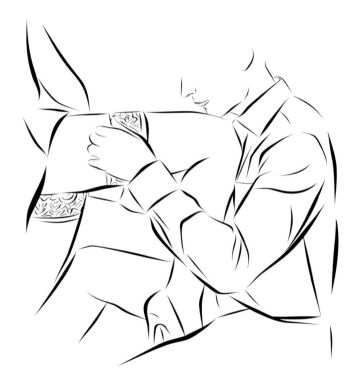

The Juliana and Clive

Hotel sex + role play = Fire emoji

Do the *Modern Family* thing and meet up at a hotel bar under new identities a la "Clive Bixby" (Phil Dunphy) and "Juliana" (Claire Dunphy.) On the show, Clive was "a business man who designs high-end electro-acoustic transducers" (hot…?) and Juliana was "a bored housewife with a dark side and an hour to kill," but you can do way better than that by creating your own alter egos.

Go ahead and invent a whole backstory. You can play by flirting as strangers OR you can go hard and do a full-on production by dressing as your characters and attending to small details like ordering something you'd never drink or wearing a different scent. Don't tell each other who you're going to be so you get to figure that out as you meet.

Arrive separately to the bar. Sit apart and make flirty eye contact first, then go up to your partner and strike up a conversation. Bring your best game because you need to lure this intriguing stranger into bed. Brush imaginary lint off their shoulder, hold your eye contact just a little bit too long, make them feel like they're the only person in the room.

If you have Dunphy money, book a hotel room ahead of time. Plan on having all your sex accoutrements, like lube, toys, birth control, and/or lingerie at the ready. Carry them in a bag or put them in the room ahead of time.

14

Bonus tip! For an extra luxe experience, book a couples' package with extras like in-room champagne or a couple's massage.

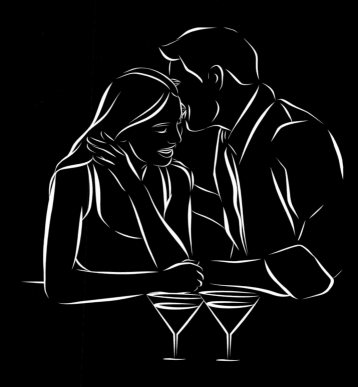

You Do Me, I Do You

15

It's nice to take turns

Turn your next toss into a game by taking turns asking each other for sexual favors.

Start the game by asking for small favors to make the game last longer and help build anticipation and lust. You might ask for a kiss or a sexy secret whispered in your ear. Gradually start sexing up the asks, zeroing in on non-dick and vulva parts. Nipple licking, neck sucking, and lubing up inner thighs are great mid-point suggestions/demands. Set a timer for each person's turn to keep it fair.

As you start getting hot and bothered, aim for suggestions that will turn you on more but won't quite get you to orgasm. The longer you can hold out, the better it will be when you finally give it. So when you follow your partner's suggestions, do what they've asked, but try not to do it *so* well that they come immediately (I know, it's hard because you're *just that good*).

When you're both beyond ready, then got ahead and ask for whatever you're craving—whether it's some of that sweet, sweet D or more of their amazing mouth or a toy fired up to full power—and let yourselves go over the edge.

This game is a great chance to discover what your partner *really* likes and for you to get exactly the kind of touch you want. Ask for things you know you love and toss in a few you might like—see what you think. Are you into a buzzy vibrator on your nipple? Maybe—find out!

15

Bonus tip! Prep your space beforehand with lube and toys and anything else that y'all might need.

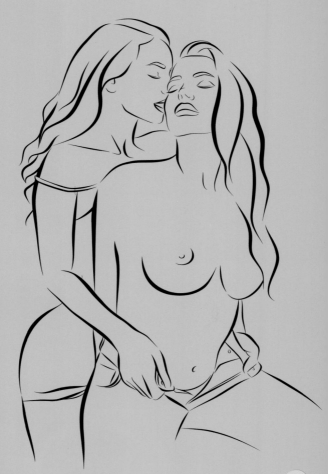

The Sex Olympics

16

You are the champions, my friend

Become contestants in your own sexual Olympics by getting a book of sex positions and trying a new one every night for a week. You can look over them together, which is its own kind of foreplay, and decide on the week's roster together. Or you can both choose a few that you want to try and the other person must do them. (Veto power allowed, but be cool about it.) Or you can leave it entirely up to fate, flip to a random page, and do whatever it is.

What if you already have a roster of positions that are reliably orgasmic? This is still definitely worth doing because A) Fun, which is good, and B) Trying new positions is a great way to discover more things you'd like to explore. If one of you keeps picking positions where they're more submissive, for example, it's not a giant leap to figure out that they might be into trying bondage or power play.

When you try a new position, especially if it's kind of hard or jacked up, approach the whole thing with a sense of fun. The point isn't to do it perfectly, or even be able to get into the position. (See also: standing positions where one person is supposed to be carrying the other one.) The point is to have a good time together. If part A doesn't get into slot B, it's still all good. And if you come up with some new favorites, even better.

16

**Bonus tip!
If you're going for
the gold medal,
do a new position
every night for a
month.**

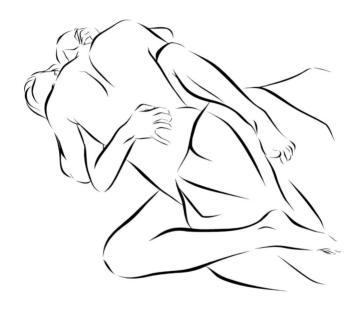

The Dessert Challenge

17

Who will be picking up the check?

Make reservations for a dinner date at a fancy restaurant. Get all dressed up. Once you get there and are seated, take turns heading to the restroom to outfit yourselves with a remote-control toy (panty vibes are a good option for vulvas, vibrating head toys work for people with penises, and butt toys work for anyone. Feel free to mix 'n match.)

When you return to the table, stealthily hand each other the remotes to the toys you're wearing. Fire up your partner's toy randomly throughout the meal. Choose toys that have different intensities and patterns so you can try out different sensations, watching to see how your partner reacts. Use the toy to take them close to orgasm, then back it up, so you can keep them in a state of anticipation and arousal. Go ahead and use your powers for evil—you do get bonus points if it's extra inappropriate, i.e., every time the waiter is at the table, turn that toy up to 11.

Keep torturing each other remotely throughout the meal. See who can keep it together until dessert. The first person to orgasm picks up the check. The best thing about this game is that there are no losers. You either get an orgasm or a free dinner.

17

Bonus tip! Choose quiet toys and a quiet table. No one needs to know what's going on down there.

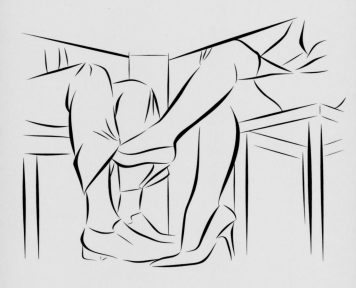

Menage a Faux

18

For when three's a crowd

Plenty of people have a fantasy about having a threesome, but only some have the desire and/or cojones to actually go through with it in real life. The solution: a fake threesome. Pretending you have a third gives you plenty of hotness with 97% less awkward interpersonal drama!

You can create the fantasy of having another person in bed with you using a few little sleights of hand (or mouth). You will also need a blindfold for whoever is getting ravished. To create the feeling of two people licking their way around your partner's body, use your own tongue, and create the feeling of another person by using a lubed finger as their "tongue."

If you're going for an extra penis, you can feign double penetration in a spoon position by sliding a penis/dildo into the bum and reaching around to slide a dildo into the vagina. If it's a bonus vagina you're looking for, straddle a partner's face with one actual vagina (or penis sleeve) while stimulating their penis with a hand vagina (lubey hands pressed together around the penis shaft to create suction and vagina-ey feel.)

This is also a great solution for couples who have one person who really, really wants a threesome and one who really, really does not. (For what it's worth, it's generally not a great idea to "give" your partner a threesome just to be a good sport.)

18

Bonus tip! If you are dramatically inclined, use a full-on different voice and personality for the "other person."

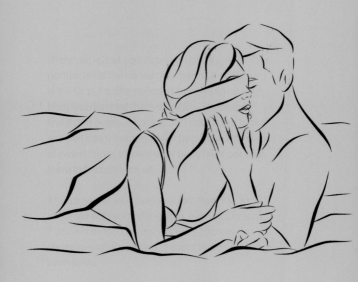

Truth or Dare

Play at your own risk

Truth or dare already has an edgy vibe to it, so lean into that with a sexed-up version. It's a great way to find out some things about each other, try out some fun/sexy dares, and generally have an adventure together. Plus, no equipment is needed, so you can bust out the game anytime.

Ideas for truths: What was it like the first time you had an orgasm? What sexual words are cringey to you? What is the kinkiest fantasy you ever had? What is your favorite fantasy to jerk off to? What was the last porn you watched? What would you like to try with me that we haven't? Have you ever seen someone else having sex, accidentally or on purpose? What is your favorite part of my body and why? What is your favorite thing I do to you? What was the hottest text/photo I ever sent you?

Ideas for dares: Play the rest of the game naked. Pretend you work at a phone sex line and answer my call. Put on my underwear and model it for me. Show me how you touch yourself when you're alone. Give a banana your best blow job. Give me a lap dance and try extra hard to earn a good tip. Go in the other room and send me a sexy pic. Act out how I look·and sound when I have an orgasm. Demonstrate your favorite oral technique on my hand.

19

Bonus tip!
If another couple suggests a game of Truth or Dare, yes, they are hitting on you.

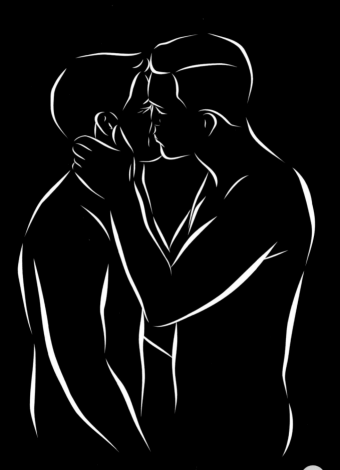

Choose Your Own Adventure

20

In case of emergency, open box

Designate a special sex box and stock it with accessories to enhance and inspire your next adventures. Fill it with whatever y'all are into (or might be into…). Plan a date night where you get to pick something out and, whatever it is, let it guide what goes down next.

For maximum fun, put stuff from a bunch of different categories in there. If lingerie is your jam, in it goes. Throw in a sexy couple's board game or card game (these do exist—try an adult store). Toss in a book of sex positions to try—open it to a page and it's on.

For sex toys, get a little something for every orifice and protrusion. Mix up stuff you know you like with stuff you maybe possibly might like. Butt toys, nipple clamps, vibrators, and dildos are good. If there is a vulva among you, toss in a clit vibrator and a G-spot toy. For penises, a penis sleeve.

Put in regular and flavored lubes and, if you're feeling brave, heating and/or cool lubes. You can also add arousal oil for penises, vulvas, and nipples. And for some CBD-infused L-O-V-E, try CBD arousal gummies, gels, or suppositories. Throw some kink in there with handcuffs or bindings, a blindfold, and a paddle, if you're feeling it.

To make it hotter, make sure you hype it up before the "Great Unboxing."

20

Bonus tip! Secretly slip something into the box, then text your partner to let them know that a new surprise present awaits them.

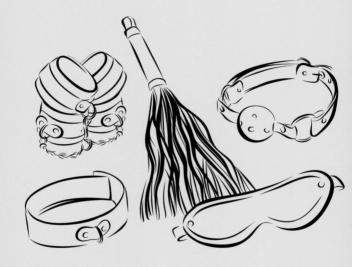

The Face Off

21

Watch and learn

Watching your partner touch themselves, and letting them watch you, is among the most intimate things you can do as a couple. Plus, it's just really f-ing hot.

Sit at opposite ends of the couch, facing each other, with your backs against each arm. Drape your legs over each other's. Squirt some lube into your hands and slide it all over your vulva/penis/whatever you've got going on. Start masturbating while you watch each other. It's like getting a private sex show, tailored specifically to you.

You can switch up the vibe by changing where you look. Try gazing into each other's eyes and watching each other as you go deeper toward orgasm. Or go ahead and stare lustfully at the other person's hand as they rub and stroke between their legs. Or if all the eye gazing is a little *too* intimate, close your eyes or stare at a neutral place like your partner's thigh or something.

Let yourselves get lost in the sensations, sounds, and visuals. Touch yourselves like you do when you're alone—not only will you get the stimulation you like, you'll be giving your partner an up-close master class on how you like to be touched. Make noise, rub as hard as you need, and if anyone wants to use a toy, no shame! The more realistic it is, the sexier it will be to both of you.

21

**Bonus tip!
If you are
competitive,
see who can have
an orgasm faster
(or slower).**

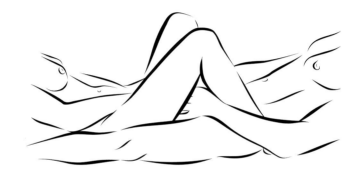

Do You Feel Me?

22

What *is* that?

Blindfold your partner—with consent, obviously—to indulge them with a session of sensory play. Start by lying them down, then brush their body with a series of objects, having them guess what each thing is.

Because they're blindfolded, your partner's other senses will be on high alert. Take advantage by playing with them with items they can feel, smell, hear, and taste. Trail a silky scarf across their chest. Brush a section of fresh peach across their mouth, dripping some juice on their lips. Take off your underwear and press it under their nose. Pop open a bottle of champagne and pour a little into their belly button. Let them hear the hum of a vibrator before you press it in their hand.

As the game progresses, sex it up by adding body parts. If you have a vulva, you could slide your wet pussy down your partner's thigh. If you're sporting a dick, try brushing your partner's lips with just the head. Tease your partner and make them ask very nicely if they'd like more of you.

You can BDSM-ify it by adding a little pain to the pleasure. (Again, enthusiastic consent mandatory.) Depending on your kink inclinations, maybe a sharp spank with a wooden spoon, a few drips of warm wax from a special candle designed for temperature play, and/or an ice cube trailing up your partner's arm.

22

**Bonus tip!
If your partner feels too vulnerable being blindfolded and lying bare-ass naked, have them lie on their stomach. Feels safer, somehow.**

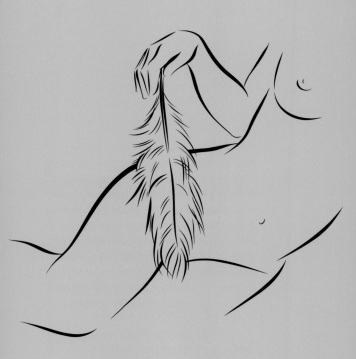

The Audition

23

Ohyeahohyeahohyeah

If both of you like porn—and "both" is key here—you can harness what you love about it by playing at being porn stars. There are a few ways to go about this.

The easiest is to put on a favorite porn and copy the moves as they're happening. Make sure you both can see the screen, then go to town. If you're a voyeur or exhibitionist, angle a big wall mirror so you can watch yourselves. (This is a great option for a hotel room when you're on vacation. There's a big bed and usually a mirror right there.) If it gets too acrobatic or you find that watching and recreating the movie at the same time is too much multitasking, just copy the sounds the actors are making.

You can also watch some porn together (it's research!), then recreate it together after. (If you have to watch it a lot to really nail those moves, so be it). This lets you combine the residual hotness of the movie with some screen-free sex where you can put the focus on each other without distraction.

If watching porn isn't really your thing, you can experiment with porn-adjacent role-play. Pretend you're acting in a movie together or make up a whole scenario. Casting director auditioning an actor for the part? One experienced porn actor teaching a newbie how to have sex onscreen? Pizza delivery gone rogue? Up to you.

23

Bonus tip! If y'all have different porn tastes, take turns being the porn DJ. Maybe you'll find something new you're into.

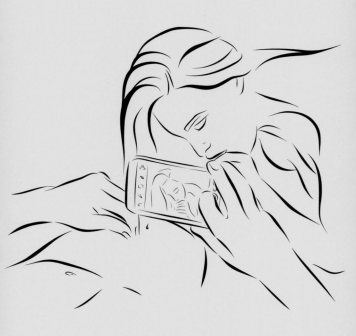

Sex Toy Gift Exchange

24

Because presents are fun

Go to a sex toy store for a naughty little shopping spree. It's retail therapy plus sex—which is 10/10, no notes—and it's also a great way to build anticipation for when you get to use those toys on each other.

You *could* order your stuff online and that's perfectly fine, but part of the whole deal is going to the store together. It's a semi-risqué adventure, plus it's a whole-ass store filled with all manner of dildos, vibrating things, silicone vaginas, pointy-looking fetish gear—it *will* get you thinking about sex.

Decide upon your mission. You can pick out a toy you want your partner to use on you or a toy to use on your partner. You could create a theme like "shower sex" and pick out stuff like waterproof toys and silicone lube, or maybe BDSM it up with a blindfold, paddle, and some handcuffs. Or pick out a couple's toy that you can use together. Shopper's choice!

After you make your selection, be sure you have whatever batteries or accessories you might need. If a toy needs a long charging before first use, make a mental note of it. A dead toy when you really need it is kind of the worst.

Once you get home, stash them away and don't let yourselves get them out to play until a predetermined special occasion. And totally okay if the special occasion is just "next Thursday." The waiting is the point.

**Bonus tip!
If you're shy/
sex store-averse,
order toys for
each other
online and
don't tell each
other what you
bought.**

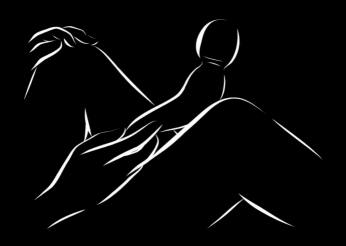

Honey Do Me Jar

25

Keep a supply of adventures on hand

Create a sex jar filled with fun ideas and y'all will always have a sexy adventure waiting for you. In a rut? Bust out the jar of sex toys—and it's on.

Here's how to do it: Both of you fill out slips of paper with sexual positions, scenarios, or other adventures you'd like to try. (About 20 each is good.) Pop 'em in a large jar. Take your time and think about what you'd *really* like.

For the safe option, write down your old favorites, like your most beloved orgasm-inducing position or recreating that certain weirdly hot time you had together (you know the one.) OR you can (should!) go ahead and try the more daring option of writing new stuff y'all have never tried, or maybe never even talked about. Maybe there's something you've been thinking about that you're not quite sure how to ask for or something you don't know if your partner would be down with. Be brave and write your *real* desires. Forty-five minutes of unreciprocated oral? In the jar! A semi-kinky thing you're kind of scared to ask for? Jar! Don't tell each other what you wrote.

When you need inspiration, pull a slip out and do whatever it says, right then, no further discussion. (Give yourselves both veto power if something sounds sketchy. But use this power sparingly.)

25 Bonus tip! If you don't know what you want (or don't want to accept responsibility), google "sex bucket list" and put the top 30 in, no questions asked.

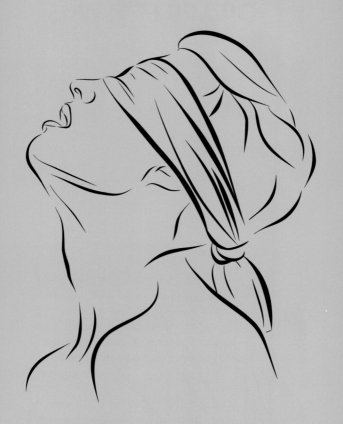

DIV BDSM

26

Your house may already be a sex dungeon

If you get the uncontrollable urge to have a BDSM session but don't have the gear, MacGyver it. There are all kinds of regular old items already lying around in your house just waiting for you to kink them out.

Don't have a blindfold? A sleep mask is just as good. Or you can tie a t-shirt, yoga pants, or scarf around your partner's head to cover their eyes. For restraints, try belts, ties, panty hose, or masking tape. (Keep scissors handy in case someone needs a quick escape.) Masking tape can double as a way to bind someone's wrists together or you can use it cover someone's mouth. There are tons of items that can be perved-out to become a paddle, including a kitchen spatula, wooden spoon, ping pong racket, fly swatter, or a hairbrush.

Did you spend your nipple clamp budget on the boring regular bills? Bust out the paper clips, clothespins, or a magnetic refrigerator clip. For temperature play, try ice cubes straight from the freezer, a warm washcloth, or a hand warmer from a dollar store. For sensation play, you can use a feather duster, a hair brush, nubby garden gloves or whatever else looks decently sexy. If something has an interesting texture and isn't harmful, give it a go. Just watch for sharp edges, splinters, and things that might break.

26

Bonus tip! If you want to add to your collection on the cheap, a dollar store has tons of instant gear like feather dusters, clothespins, and hand warmers.

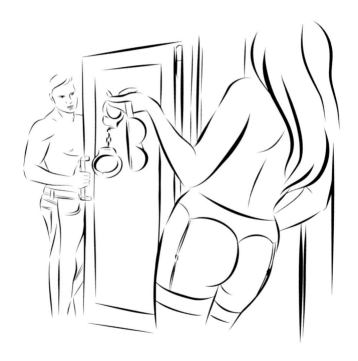

Tantric Lite

27

Oh-ohhhhhmmmm

Tantra is an ancient Indian practice that's about much more than sex, but you can skip the meditation and yoga and just borrow some of it for sex. No one needs to know.

For six nights, have sex (whatever that means to you) as much as you want, but without orgasms. A good way to start a session is to sit facing each other. Put your hands on each other's hearts, gaze into each other's eyes, and sync your breathing. When you feel connected, start slowly touching each other, focusing on every sensation.

Try to get to a space of uber-mindfulness where you can let yourself really focus on each other and the pleasure of touching each other without any sort of goal. Because no one's expecting an orgasm, it's a lot easier to relax into the experience and linger in that sexual space with each other. Take the time to explore each other's bodies. Don't have a plan, just see where it all takes you.

Try to draw out the experience as long as possible. If you're having penetrative sex, you could lie together for several long moments, enjoying the feeling of having someone inside you/being inside your partner. Or you could give each other oral, but a really slow version that makes every lick feel incredible.

On day seven, it's orgasm day. Or… maybe you'll want to keep it going. Up to you and your fiery loins.

27

Bonus tip! If it takes you a while to get turned on, try a solo tantric session before you see your partner.

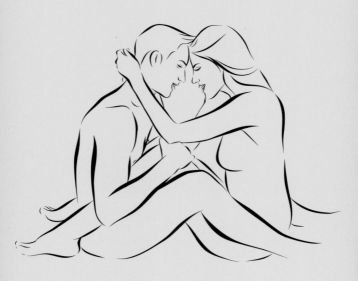

Guess the Sex Toy

What is touching me?
Dunno, you'll have to guess.

Anything that focuses your attention on the moment and whatever sensations are happening is gonna sexy up your sex. If that "anything" is a sex toy, hey, even better. And sex toys, plural? C'mon! It's going to be good. Real good.

To start, lie your partner on their back and blindfold them. Have an array of different types of toys at the ready. Depending on what equipment people are sporting, add a clit vibrator, a penis sleeve, and/or a prostrate toy. G-spot vibes work for both vaginas and prostrates. (Just don't switch from butt to vagina to keep bacteria out. The reverse—vagina to butt—is okay though.) Wand vibes can be used all over the body.

Start by running toys along your partner's non-genital areas, like arms, legs, the palms of their hands, and so on. As you go along, intensify it by letting a vibe linger on their vulva or the base of their penis. If you're going to penetrate your partner with a toy, this would be the time.

Go ahead and use the "wrong" toys on each other. A clitoral suction vibe on a nipple? Could work. A swishy penis sleeve lubed up and rubbed across a vulva? Sure. A dildo brushed across your partner's lips? Why the F not?

Did they guess all the toys? Doesn't matter, you both still win.

28

Bonus tip! To help your partner feel less vulnerable, always keep a hand on their body to anchor them and let them know you're there.

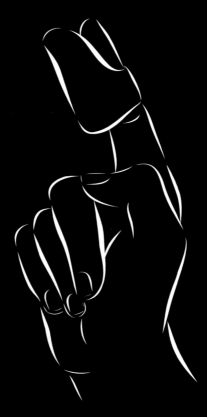

Where's Your Honey?

29

The best honey do list ever

Give your partner a good reason to trail their tongue all over your body with a private tasting session. Blindfold your partner (with consent, as with all blindfolding situations). Put a dollop of sweet honey somewhere on your body. Ask your partner to find the sweetness using just their mouth—no hands allowed.

Start with honey on your finger, the crook of your arm or the little divot in your neck. (It's called the suprasternal notch. Maybe don't bring up this highly interesting fact during the game.) Then put the honey in places where you need their mouth, like your lips, nipples, or between your legs. (Caveat: Don't actually put sugary stuff *in* the vagina. It will muck about with pH levels, which is not good.)

There are lots of variations you can try. After your partner finds the honey (yay them!), it's your turn to try. Or put a little dollop of something on your body but don't tell them what it is. They get to find it and guess what it is. You could also make yourself into a human buffet by putting little dabs of sweet things all over your body all at once for them to find and lick off.

If honey is not your partner's jam, feel free to sub it out with something else, even actual jam if you want. You can also try whipped cream, chocolate syrup, berries, peanut butter, or even sushi.

29

Bonus tip! Put some old towels or sheets down because it's gonna get messy.

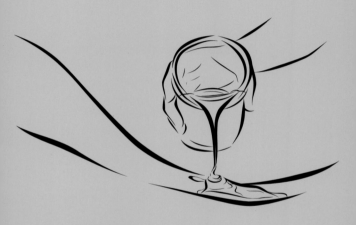

The Buildup

30

Go really deep with each other

Sensate focus is a technique therapists use to help their clients feel closer and less anxious. And you can definitely use it for that—it's great if one or both of you have trouble getting out of your head during sex—but you can also use it to make your sex feel more intimate and urgent.

Try the method over four nights. You can do four in a row, or make a weekly date. For the first night, you take turns stroking, kissing, and massaging the other person's body. On day one, there's no touching of breasts or genitals. This is one-way touch only. The receiver's only job is to lie back and notice the feeling and emotions that come up. Set a timer for 10 to 15 minutes, then trade.

On day two, it's still one-way touch, with a designated giver and receiver, but you can add boobs and dicks/vulvas. You're not going for an orgasm here (at least not yet), you're just exploring how it feels to touch and be touched.

For day three, it's mutual touch. You can touch, kiss, and stroke each other anywhere, but don't do anything that will lead to orgasm. Again, you're just connecting, feeling, and exploring.

On the fourth night, it's on. You get the green light on oral, hand jobs, penetrative sex, whatever you want. But instead of just jumping each other, keep your heightened focus going and really enjoy every touch.

30

Bonus tip! This is definitely the time to bust out the candlelight and sexy music.

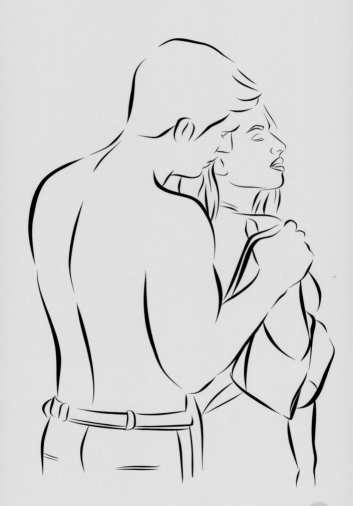